GET FIT IN NO TIME

Easy Home Exercises for Seniors Over 60

Janet martins

Contents

DISCLAIMER:

All content is provided as general information only, and should not be taken as medical advice or professional guidance. Please consult with a qualified healthcare provider if you have any questions or concerns about your individual situation.

INTRODUCTION

Are you over 60 searching for ways to get fit without leaving home? Look no further! We have compiled a list of easy home exercises designed for seniors to help you hit your fitness goals in no time! Whether you are looking to improve your strength, balance, or flexibility – these simple exercises are perfect for anyone wanting to live a healthier lifestyle. So, don't delay and start getting fit today!

Being over 60 doesn't mean you have to let go of all physical activity! But, with simple home exercises for seniors, you can get fit and stay active in no time! There are a variety of easy-to-follow routines and exercises that can help those over sixty maintain their health and well-being without the need for expensive equipment or gym memberships. So, whether you're just starting out or simply looking for an effective way to stay in shape, these easy home exercises for seniors will help you reach your fitness goals!

Staying physically active is essential for everyone, but it is particularly important for seniors. A sedentary lifestyle can affect your health in many ways, from increased risk of heart disease to decreased mobility and depression. Fortunately, it's never too late to start exercising! With the right home exercises for seniors over 60, you can get fit in no time and start feeling better about yourself and your daily life.

PART 1

WHAT IS AN EXERCISE

Exercise the training of the body to improve its function and enhance its fitness.

Exercise and physical activity are often used interchangeably, but this article will distinguish between them. Physical activity is an inclusive term that refers to any expenditure of energy brought about by bodily movement via the skeletal muscles; as such, it includes the complete spectrum of activity from very low resting levels to maximal exertion. Exercise is a component of physical activity. The distinguishing characteristic of exercise is that it is a structured activity specifically planned to develop and maintain physical fitness. Physical conditioning refers to the development of physical fitness through the adaptation of the body and its various systems to an exercise program.

Exercise is also known as physical activity. In simple terms, exercise is any movement that works your body at a greater intensity than your usual level of daily activity. Exercise raises your heart rate and works your muscles and is most commonly undertaken to achieve the aim of physical fitness.

Exercise is a physical activity that is planned, structured, and repetitive for the purpose of conditioning the body. The exercise consists of cardiovascular conditioning, strength and resistance training, and flexibility.

BENEFITS OF EXERCISE

So what are the benefits of regular exercise? Not only can it give you more energy, but it can also improve your mood, help you sleep better and live longer (to name a few). Here are some reasons why exercise is so important.

Makes you feel happier

Who doesn't love the rush of endorphins after a brisk walk or spin class?

Endorphins are hormones that reduce pain and boost pleasure, creating a general feeling of well-being and positivity. So before you roll your eyes at your enthusiastic fitness instructor, consider how a steady state of endorphins does the body good.

Endorphins also act as a natural painkiller and can help ease long-term aches. In addition, regular exercise can strengthen muscles, lessening chronic pain and your risk of injury.

Gives you more energy

Physical activity increases your heart rate and gets your blood flowing. Likewise, more oxygen and nutrients to your muscles mean higher energy levels. And although it seems odd that expending energy can give you more energy, science backs this claim up.

One study found that 90% of people who completed a regular exercise program reported improved fatigue compared to those who did not exercise. So next time you're considering an extra cup of coffee to perk you up, try a walk instead.

Promotes quality sleep

Exercise can reduce stress and anxiety levels, leaving you feeling more relaxed and stabilized, which is a perfect zone for sleep.

And while working out can also raise your body temperature and make you feel more alert throughout the day, it can also help you drift off better when your internal temperature starts to dip back down.

If you exercise outside, exposure to vitamin D can also regulate your wake-sleep cycle. Just tread carefully with when you work out and how close it is to bedtime.

Helps fight depression

Research shows that for mild or moderate cases of depression, exercise can be an effective treatment.

Exercising increases your brain's sensitivity to serotonin and norepinephrine, which ease feelings of depression.

But you can skip training for a marathon to gain the benefits.

One study showed that just six weeks of yoga (in addition to standard treatment) was enough to reduce depression and even anxiety. Yoga and Pilates also focus on breathing exercises, which can reduce stress and promote relaxation.

Helps maintain strong muscles and bones

As we get older, we lose muscle mass and function. But exercising regularly may reduce muscle loss and maintain strength. As we exercise, our bodies release hormones that help muscles absorb amino acids and boost muscle growth.

And according to a study, exercising while we're young helps build bone density, which can help prevent osteoporosis as we age.

Reduces risk of chronic disease

Exercising regularly can help ward off chronic diseases like Type 2 diabetes and heart disease. It can also help if you have high blood pressure and high cholesterol.

Just think about how a lack of exercise can impact your health. It can cause significant belly fat (which we know is tough to lose) and has been linked to high cholesterol, inflammation, heart disease, stroke, and diabetes.

Reduces pain

If you have chronic low back pain, fibromyalgia, or other conditions that cause chronic pain, exercising has been shown to help reduce pain.

Research shows that exercise can reduce the severity of pain, as well as improve physical function.

Boosts your brain health

Exercise is beneficial for maintaining brain health for everyone, but even more for those at risk for developing dementia and Alzheimer's disease.

Movement promotes cardiovascular health, improves blood flow to the brain, and reduces inflammation. It also stimulates the production of hormones that enhance the growth of brain cells.

A study suggests that exercise can also impact the hippocampus in older adults. This part of the brain is important for memory and learning.

Exercise can help it grow, which may improve mental function.

Improves skin

With the sweat that comes from working out, you may not think that exercise can positively impact your skin. But regular moderate exercise may increase antioxidants in your body.

Those antioxidants help protect cells from oxidative stress and free radicals, which can damage your skin.

Exercising also increases blood flow which can help with anti-aging effects.

Improves sex life

Exercise can lead to a stronger heart and muscles and improve flexibility, which can benefit your sex life.

Research also shows that in postmenopausal women who exercised, their sexual desire increased, while exercise significantly improved erectile function in men.

Helps maintain weight

If you're at your ideal weight, exercising can help in a variety of ways. In addition to using excess calories stored as fat, working out helps maintain muscle mass and repair muscles.

It also reduces stress and can help you sleep — all of which lead to good choices when it comes to eating.

Helps you live longer

Healthcare providers recommend regular exercise to improve or prevent conditions like diabetes, heart disease, some forms of cancer, and obesity.

But it also keeps your bones, muscles, and joints healthy, lowers cholesterol and blood pressure, and protects your mental health. All of these amazing benefits can add up to one thing living longer (plus feeling good).

TYPES OF EXERCISE

1. Aerobic exercise

Aerobic exercise speeds up your heart rate and breathing and is important for many body functions. It gives your heart and lungs a workout and increases endurance. "If you're too winded to walk up a flight of stairs, that's a good indicator that you need more aerobic exercise to help condition your heart and lungs and get enough blood to your muscles to help them work efficiently," says Wilson.

Aerobic exercise also helps relax blood vessel walls, lower blood pressure, burn body fat, lower blood sugar levels, reduce inflammation, boost mood, and raise "good" HDL cholesterol. In addition, it can lower "bad" LDL cholesterol levels, combined with weight loss. Over the long term, aerobic exercise reduces your risk of heart disease, stroke, type 2 diabetes, breast and colon cancer, depression, and falls.

Aim for 150 minutes per week of moderate-intensity activity. For example, try brisk walking, swimming, jogging, cycling, dancing, or classes like step aerobics.

Starting position: Stand tall with your feet together and arms at your sides.

Movement: Bend your elbows and swing your arms as you lift your knees.

March in a variety of styles:

- March is in place.
- March four steps forward, and then four steps back.
- March in place with feet wide apart.

- Alternate marching feet wide and together (out, out, in, in).

Tips and techniques:

- Look straight ahead and keep your abs tight.
- Breathe comfortably, and don't clench your fists.

Make it easier: March slower, and don't lift your knees as high.

Make it harder: Lift your knees higher, march faster, and pump your arms.

1. Strength training

As we age, we lose muscle mass. Strength training builds it back. "Regular strength training will help you feel more confident and capable of daily tasks like carrying groceries, gardening, and lifting heavier objects around the house. Strength training will also help you stand up from a chair, get off the floor, and go upstairs," says Wilson.

Strengthening your muscles makes you stronger and stimulates bone growth, lowers blood sugar, assists with weight control, improves balance and posture, and reduces stress and pain in the lower back and joints.

Starting position: Stand with your feet shoulder-width apart, arms at your sides.

Movement:

1. Slowly bend your hips and knees, lowering your buttocks about eight inches, as if sitting back in a chair.
2. Let your arms swing forward to help you balance.
3. Keep your back straight.
4. Slowly return to the starting position.

5. Repeat 8-12 times.

Tips and techniques:

- Shift your weight into your heels.
- Squeeze your buttocks as you stand to help you balance.

Make it easier:

1. Sit on the edge of a chair with your feet hip-width apart and arms crossed over your chest.
2. Tighten your abdominal muscles and stand up.
3. Slowly sit down with control.

Make it harder: Lower farther, but not past your thighs being parallel to the floor.

1. Stretching

Stretching helps maintain flexibility. We often overlook that in youth when our muscles are healthier. But aging leads to a loss of flexibility in the muscles and tendons. Muscles shorten and don't function properly. That increases the risk of muscle cramps and pain, muscle damage, strains, joint pain, and falling, and it also makes it tough to get through daily activities, such as bending down to tie your shoes.

Likewise, stretching the muscles routinely makes them longer and more flexible, which increases your range of motion and reduces pain and the risk of injury.

Starting position: Lie on your back with your legs on the floor.

Movement:

1. Relax your shoulders against the floor.

2. Bend your left knee and place your left foot on your right thigh just above the knee.

3. Tighten your abdominal muscles, grasp your left knee with your right hand, and

gently pull it across your body toward your right side.

Hold for 10 to 30 seconds.

Return to the starting position and repeat on the other side.

Tips and techniques:

- Stretch to the point of mild tension, not pain.
- Try to keep both shoulders flat on the floor.
- To increase the stretch, look in the direction opposite to your knee.

1. Balance exercises

Improving your balance makes you feel steadier and helps prevent falls. It's especially important as we get older when the systems that help us maintain balance, our vision, our inner ear, and our leg muscles and joints tend to break down.

The good news is that training your balance can help prevent and reverse these losses," says Wilson.

Many senior centers and gyms offer balance-focused exercise classes, such as tai chi or yoga. It's always early enough to start this exercise, even if you don't have balance problems.

Starting position: Stand up straight with your feet together and your hands on your hips.

Movement: Lift your left knee toward the ceiling as high as is comfortable or until your thigh is parallel to the floor. Hold, then slowly lower your knee to the starting position.

Repeat the exercise 3-5 times.

Then perform the exercise 3-5 times with your right leg.

Tips and techniques:

- Keep your chest lifted and your shoulders down and back.
- Lift your arms to your sides to help you balance, if needed.
- Tighten your abdominal muscles throughout.
- Tighten the buttock of your standing leg for stability.
- Breathe comfortably.

Make it easier: Hold on to the back of a chair or counter with one hand.

Make it harder: Lower your leg to the floor without touching it. Just as it is about to touch, lift your leg again.

WHY IS EXERCISE IMPORTANT FOR SENIORS OVER 60

1. Maintains independent living – This is perhaps the main benefit of exercising into older age. While care homes are essential for some, many older adults would like to live independently for as long as possible. Therefore, maintaining an exercise regimen that supports this lifestyle is vital.

2. Better cardiovascular health – Physical activity for adults and older adults reduces the risk of cardiovascular disease by 35%. Heart attacks and strokes are medical conditions that, if survived, often result in life-altering consequences. Exercise can, therefore, be a huge preventative intervention.

3. May assist cognitive function – Dementia affects many older adults, with the Alzheimers Society indicating there are predicted to be over 1 million people with the condition by 2025. Some studies have suggested that exercise is a measure that may help reduce the incidence of the disease.

4. Reduces anxiety and depression – Many older adults may face social withdrawal, illness, or disability, any of which can result in mental health issues. Exercise has a range of cognitive benefits, with studies showing that it reduces anxiety and depression, boasting a significant reduction in relapse compared to other interventions.

5. Helps with flexibility – Osteoarthritic pain poses a significant issue for older adults, with joints and muscles becoming stiff and immobile. While an exercise regimen can't reverse all age-related joint changes, maintaining movement in muscles and joints is essential to decrease discomfort.

6. Improves strength – Muscles waste without exercise. In the same way that movement improves flexibility, the right resistance training strengthens important muscle groups to keep you independently mobile. This is especially useful when going from sitting to standing, up and down stairs, or walking.

7. Improves bone density – Many older adults have osteoporosis, where bones weaken and become more susceptible to fractures. Performing regular resistance training is proven to maintain bone strength in later years.

8. Prevents falls – Falls are a significant risk when people lose flexibility, strength, and coordination. Other risk factors might also include illness or disability. Exercise can reduce the risk of falls, injuries, and potential hospital admissions.

9. Maintains hobbies – If an individual loses the ability to participate in activities due to inactivity, it can have negative physical and psychological repercussions. Hobbies are essential to remaining socially connected and engaged in life.

10. Assists weight loss – Diet and inactivity can contribute to weight gain in later years, resulting in a higher incidence of associated medical conditions. Exercise is a calorie-burning activity and can encourage you to pursue a healthier diet. Furthermore, physical activity can reduce the likelihood of Type Two Diabetes by up to 40%.

11. Forms a cornerstone habit – Exercise is a habit that behavioral scientists have shown to facilitate other productive routines, such as healthy eating and social interaction. Physical activity can, therefore, have a host of positive knock-on effects.

12. Improves sleep – Getting enough sleep has been demonstrated to reduce the incidence of chronic physical and mental health conditions and is, therefore, essential for our emotional well-being. In addition, exercise can help reduce mental activity as well as induce physical fatigue, assisting sleep patterns.

13. Sustains social connections – When performed in a social environment, exercise keeps you accountable and is hugely rewarding. Whether that's an exercise class at the local leisure center or a regular walk in the park with a friend, reinforcing social bonds is vital to good health in later years.

14. Increases confidence – More than simply the physical benefits of exercise, regular movement and training can be confidence boosting, nourishing the mind-body connection. Moreover, higher self-esteem through exercise can boost happiness and a greater quality of life in later years.

15. Increases lifespan – Studies have demonstrated that regular exercise can add 3-5 years to life expectancy figures. Physical activity not only adds years but improves the quality of those years.

16. It's fun! Why do children play games? They don't consider the exercise benefits but regard movement as its reward. Although you might find it hard to return to exercise after a long absence, you'll soon enjoy the progress as your fitness and mobility levels improve.

If you have a medical condition or are unsure what type of physical activity is appropriate, it's best to consult your GP or physiotherapist before exercising.

PART 2:

GETTING STARTED WITH EXERCISE

FINDING AN APPROPRIATE WORKOUT PLAN FOR SENIORS

Exercising regularly is crucial to maintaining good health as a senior. But it's important to find the right exercise plan - one that is safe, tailored to your needs and abilities, and enjoyable enough to motivate you to stick with it.

Consult a doctor or physical therapist who can guide you on what workout plan might work best for you. They may also recommend certain exercises or classes specifically designed for seniors.

No matter what type of workout plan you decide is right for you, it should include some combination of aerobic activity (such as walking or swimming), strength training, flexibility exercises, and balance activities. To ensure you're doing the exercises correctly and safely, look for a certified instructor or physical therapist who can supervise.

It's also important to start slowly and increase the intensity gradually over time. Start with shorter sessions and work to longer workout times as you get more comfortable with the exercises. Lastly, don't forget to take breaks when needed – it's OK if you need to rest between sets or take days off from exercising.

By finding the right exercise plan that works best for you, seniors can stay active, healthy, and independent well into their golden years.

1 . Create a personalized plan with your doctor or physical therapist

2 . Look for exercise classes designed for seniors

3 . Consider a combination of aerobic, strength, flexibility, and balance activities

4. Start slowly and increase the intensity gradually

5. Take breaks when needed to avoid injury and fatigue

6 . Stay active, healthy, and independent by exercising regularly

TIPS TO STAY MOTIVATED AND CONSISTENT

FIND SOMETHING YOU ENJOY DOING.

I'm not a huge fan of the phrase "exercise isn't fun" because there are so many activities out there that are both a good workout and fun!

Maybe you hate going to the gym but love walking the track with a friend. Or you would love a good strength workout with weights. Or a fitness class is more your style!

Plus, consider all the other possibilities aside from what we traditionally consider exercise. For example, could you do a trampoline workout? Take a pole dancing class? Go hiking with friends?

There are so many possibilities to find the joyful movement that you love. Find one!

SCHEDULE YOUR WORKOUTS INTO YOUR PLANNER.

If you get to the end of the week and realize you haven't managed to 'fit in' a workout, try scheduling them in your planner. And then stick with that scheduled item just like any other priority in your calendar!

This is good because it forces you to look ahead at the week to see where you can fit in exercise time, which makes you more likely to stick with it.

SET SPECIFIC GOALS.

If you say, "I want to exercise more," — that's a big, overarching goal. Break it down to be more specific. How many days per week? How many minutes? What will you be doing?

For example, what training plan will you use if you want to train for a half marathon? What date will you start? What days of the week will you run?

Setting specific goals you help yourself stay more accountable and provides a measurable framework to assess your progress.

SIGN UP FOR SOMETHING.

I'm a runner and triathlete, so my 'go-to' task when feeling unmotivated is to sign up for a race. It puts a definitive goal on the calendar, and by paying for it, I am committed.

But running and triathlons aren't for everyone, and that's OK. So if racing isn't your thing, consider something else you could sign up for to keep you on track.

Paying for ten Zumba classes (rather than the class-by-class drop-in fee) will encourage you to attend classes more frequently. Or you feel you'd mesh with a new personal trainer at the gym, and you can sign up for a personal training session.

FIND A FITNESS FRIEND.

Enlist the help of a spouse, friend, or coworker who loves exercising, and set up times to work out together. Accountability and friendship are great tools for sticking to your goals. Plus, if you're competitive, you may push yourself more when exercising with a partner.

USE THE 10-MINUTE RULE.

Wear your workout clothes and sneakers and commit to doing just 10 minutes. If you feel like going home after that, go ahead. But most of the time, you'll see the hardest part was getting out the door – once you're there, you'll probably want to continue.

CONSIDER USING FITNESS APPS.

Tons of fitness apps might be useful for you, whether for accountability or motivation. I've

Setting specific goals you help yourself stay more accountable and provides a measurable framework to assess your progress.

SIGN UP FOR SOMETHING.

I'm a runner and triathlete, so my 'go-to' task when feeling unmotivated is to sign up for a race. It puts a definitive goal on the calendar, and by paying for it, I am committed.

But running and triathlons aren't for everyone, and that's OK. So if racing isn't your thing, consider something else you could sign up for to keep you on track.

Paying for ten Zumba classes (rather than the class-by-class drop-in fee) will encourage you to attend classes more frequently. Or you feel you'd mesh with a new personal trainer at the gym, and you can sign up for a personal training session.

FIND A FITNESS FRIEND.

Enlist the help of a spouse, friend, or coworker who loves exercising, and set up times to work out together. Accountability and friendship are great tools for sticking to your goals. Plus, if you're competitive, you may push yourself more when exercising with a partner.

USE THE 10-MINUTE RULE.

Wear your workout clothes and sneakers and commit to doing just 10 minutes. If you feel like going home after that, go ahead. But most of the time, you'll see the hardest part was getting out the door – once you're there, you'll probably want to continue.

CONSIDER USING FITNESS APPS.

Tons of fitness apps might be useful for you, whether for accountability or motivation. I've come across a few, but this is just a quick glance – there are tons out there.

ADD SOME NEW TUNES – OR COMEDY!

There's just something about a new playlist that gets me pumped about working out! Those helpful tunes encourage you to push yourself and enjoy your workout.

SWITCH THINGS UP.

This goes along with the tip about finding something you love but is more specifically towards those who enjoy the activity – but need a little bit of boredom busted.

GET IT DONE FIRST THING IN THE MORNING.

Let's first set the record straight – the best time of day to work out is whatever time works for you. But if you frequently skip the post-work sweat sessions, consider starting a morning workout routine instead.

Try setting that alarm an hour earlier a few days a week. Getting it done and out of the way will have you feeling fabulous.

PART 3:

SAFETY CONSIDERATIONS FOR SENIORS EXERCISING

1. Go At An Easy Pace

When exercising, encourage your loved one to go slow and space out each activity. Allow your loved one to take breaks between sessions. Failing to stop and rest could increase the risk of a heart attack, stroke, and other cardiovascular issues. Going too hard in the gym and overworking the muscles can also increase the risk of broken bones and fractures. One of the best ways to avoid exerting too much energy is to set realistic and achievable goals.

2. Eat Healthily

Many seniors are afraid to eat before exercising because they fear the food will make them sluggish and sleepy. However, when the body gets the vitamins, minerals, and nutrients it needs, metabolism increases and provides more energy while working out, which also lowers the risk of accidents and injuries. So your loved one should consume healthy calories before exercising instead of unhealthy foods like cookies, cakes, candies, and sugary beverages.

3. Choose Water-Based Exercises

Low-impact activities like water aerobics are safe for seniors because the buoyancy from the water puts less stress on the body, even for adults with weaker muscles. In the water, seniors can move around with more confidence instead of worrying about falling and breaking their bones. Water also acts as a form of resistance, reducing the need to complete routines using heavy weights. When older adults take up water-based exercises, they're more likely to remain active due to the safety benefits associated with these activities.

4. Use Supportive Devices

Your loved one may need to lean on a chair or wall when exercising to prevent an accident or injury. Encourage your loved one to use medical devices if he or she has mobility limitations or cognitive issues that affect balance and flexibility. Also, make the activity easier based on your loved one's skills. For example, if your loved one uses a cane to walk around, find ways to exercise while sitting down. Your loved one can use a chair or bench to avoid falling when working out.

A professional caregiver can provide support for your loved one during exercise to prevent falls. There are many reasons seniors might need assistance at home. Some may require regular mental stimulation due to an Alzheimer's diagnosis, while others might only need part-time assistance with exercise and basic household tasks. Home Care Assistance is a leading homecare provider. Families rely on our expertly trained caregivers to help their senior loved ones maintain a high quality of life.

5. Stay Hydrated

Aging causes the amount of water in the body to decrease, putting seniors at a higher risk of dehydration. Proper hydration is necessary to lubricate the joints and regulate body temperature. Your loved one should drink plenty of liquids before, during, and after a workout and consume healthy foods that contain water, such as cucumbers, broccoli, spinach, and apples. Staying hydrated reduces the risk of fainting or falling while exercising.

MODIFYING THE EXERCISE PROGRAM FOR MOBILITY LIMITATIONS

For seniors with mobility limitations, modifying the exercise program to their individual needs and abilities is important. Activities such as yoga, tai chi, swimming, and walking are great low-impact exercises that can be adapted for any physical level.

When starting a new exercise routine or adapting an existing one, seniors should always consult their doctor first. It is also helpful to work with a certified fitness instructor who can provide modifications based on the senior's specific abilities. He/she can also provide assistance in creating a safe and effective workout plan tailored to the individual's needs and capabilities.

Regular physical activity has many benefits for seniors over 60. Exercise helps maintain strength, balance, flexibility, and overall health - all of which are key for maintaining independence and quality of life. With the right modifications, seniors can enjoy a safe, effective exercise program that will help them stay fit and healthy.

BENEFITS OF INCORPORATING EXERCISE INTO DAILY ACTIVITIES.

Provides Consistency

A consistent workout plan helps build endurance and leads to better sleep quality, less stress, and an improved mood. According to Healthline, a study in which 26 healthy men and women who exercised regularly and were asked to continue or stop their workouts for two weeks showed that "those who stopped exercising experienced increases in a negative mood.

You're also less likely to fall off the exercise wagon when you incorporate a fitness plan into your daily schedule. Adding it to your routine becomes a realistic part of your life. Choose specific days and times for your physical activity and stick to them. You'll no longer have to worry about finding time to exercise if it's already on your to-do list.

Achieves Work-Life Balance

When you have a good fitness plan, you're less likely to feel conflicted between your personal life and your work life. According to The Huffington Post, consistent exercise boosts your self-efficacy and the confidence to get things done. In addition, it helps you attain the physical and mental endurance you need to persevere daily.

Saint Leo University management professor, Russell Clayton, discussed his research findings of a positive relationship between physical activity and work-home life management.

Provides Structure and Discipline

A workout schedule sets guidelines and expectations leading to a better, structured life. Everything is laid out for you so you're not wondering what to do next and, in turn, save time for other things on your to-do list.

Keeping up with your fitness will also help you become more disciplined. As a result, you'll find yourself having more control of your day with a stronger focus on accomplishing your goals.

CONCLUSION

There are many benefits to exercising regularly for seniors over 60, including increased strength, improved balance, and increased flexibility. Exercise can also help keep bones and joints healthy. Even just a few minutes of light exercise per day can make a big difference in overall health. For seniors over 60 who want to improve their health and mobility, incorporating regular physical activity into their routine is essential. Taking the time to engage in daily physical activity can pay off in better health now and down the road.

By staying active throughout life, seniors over 60 can enjoy an improved quality of life that includes greater mental clarity and energy levels while reducing the risk of chronic diseases such as heart disease and diabetes. Exercise helps people stay independent longer by keeping mobility and strength at an optimal level. Taking the time to exercise now can help ensure a healthy future.

The key is to find enjoyable activities that work for each individual's lifestyle and physical abilities. With guidance and support from a doctor or certified fitness professional, seniors over 60 can develop an exercise program tailored to their needs and goals. Regular physical activity is essential for maintaining health and independence in old age, so take the time to exercise today!